In the same series by Roland Fiddy:
The Fanatic's Guide to The Bed
The Fanatic's Guide to Cats
The Fanatic's Guide to Computers
The Fanatic's Guide to Dads
The Fanatic's Guide to Diets
The Fanatic's Guide to Dogs
The Fanatic's Guide to Golf
The Fanatic's Guide to Husbands
The Fanatic's Guide to Money
The Fanatic's Guide to Sex

First published in the USA in 1992 by Exley Giftbooks
Published in Great Britain in 1992 by Exley Publications Ltd

Copyright © Roland Fiddy, 1992

ISBN 1-85015-313-2

Typeset by Brush Off Studios, St Albans, Herts AL3 4PH.
Printed in Great Britain by William Clowes Ltd, Beccles, Suffolk.

Exley Publications Ltd, 16 Chalk Hill, Watford, Herts WD1 4BN,
United Kingdom.
Exley Giftbooks, 487 East Main Street, Suite 326, Mount Kisco, NY
10549-0110, USA.

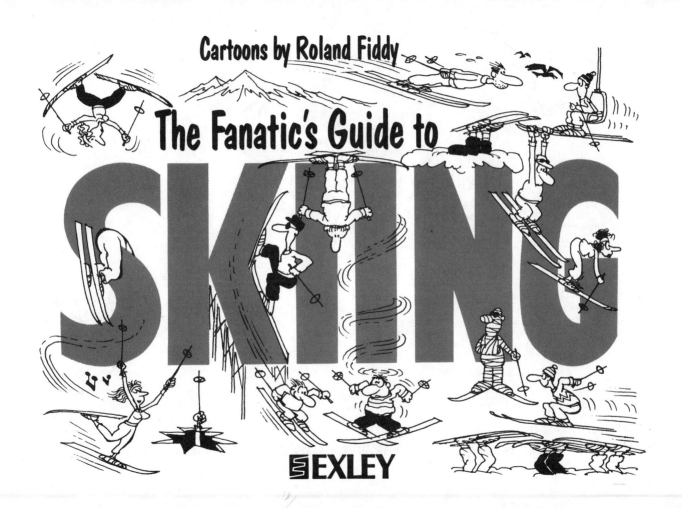

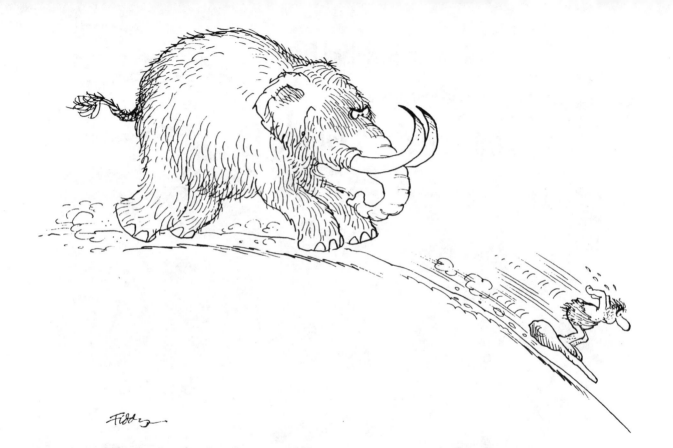

THERE IS A BASIC HUMAN URGE TO TRAVEL FASTER THAN YOUR LEGS WILL CARRY YOU...

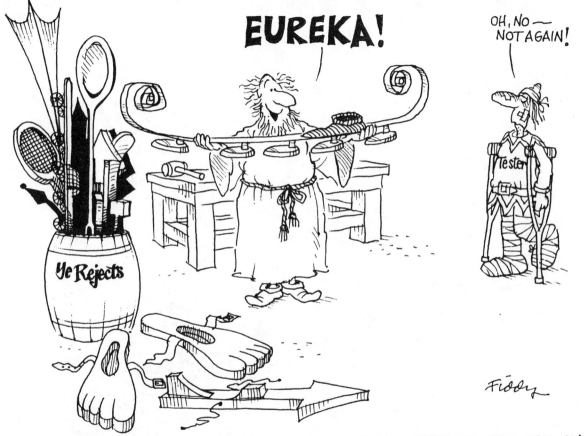

...BUT IT TOOK MANY YEARS OF TRIAL AND ERROR BEFORE THE SKI IN ITS PRESENT FORM WAS PERFECTED.

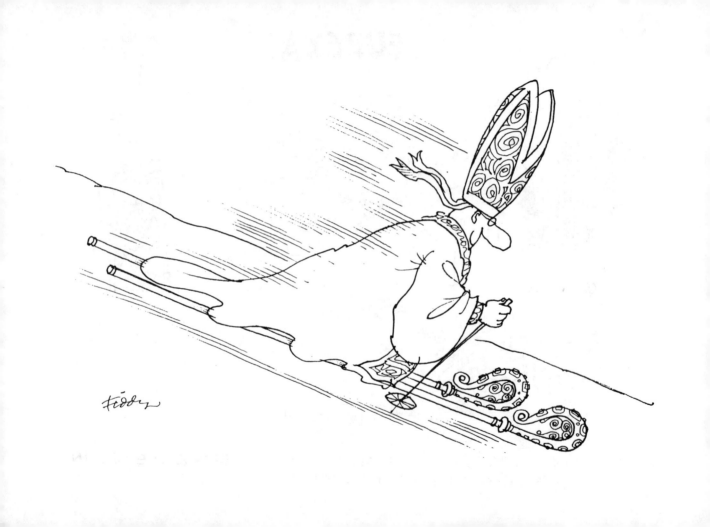

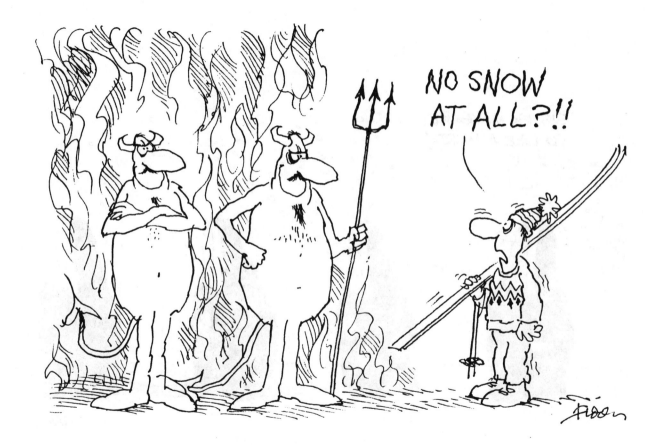

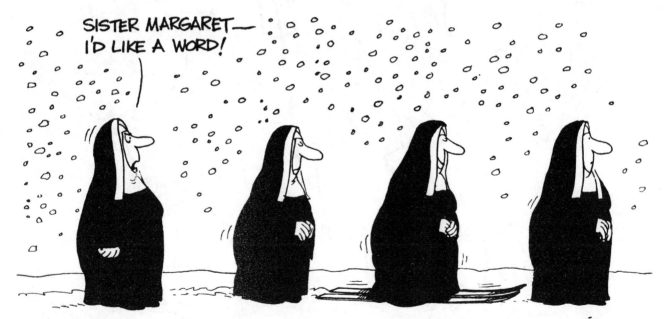

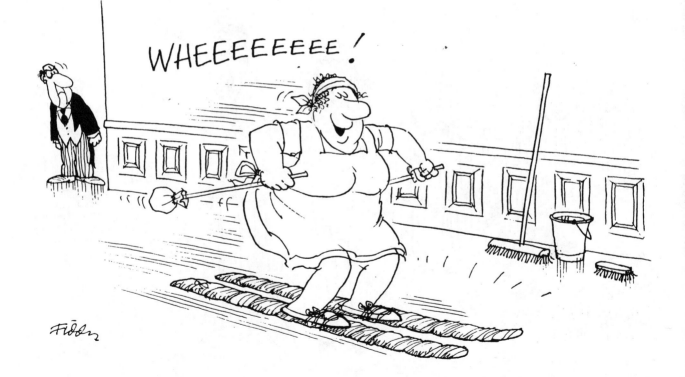

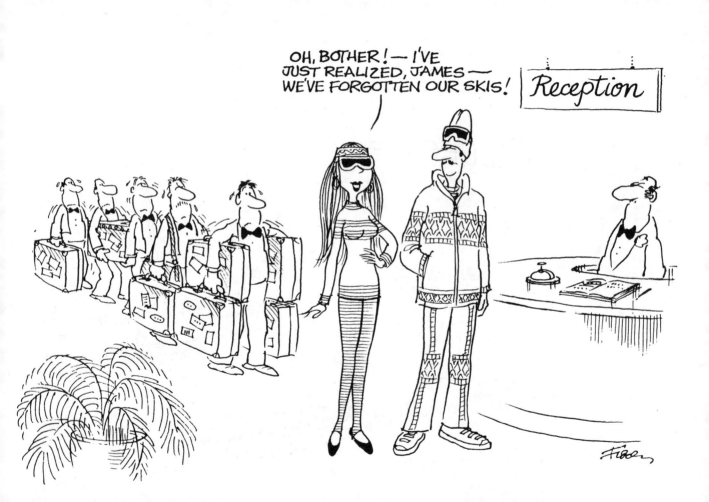

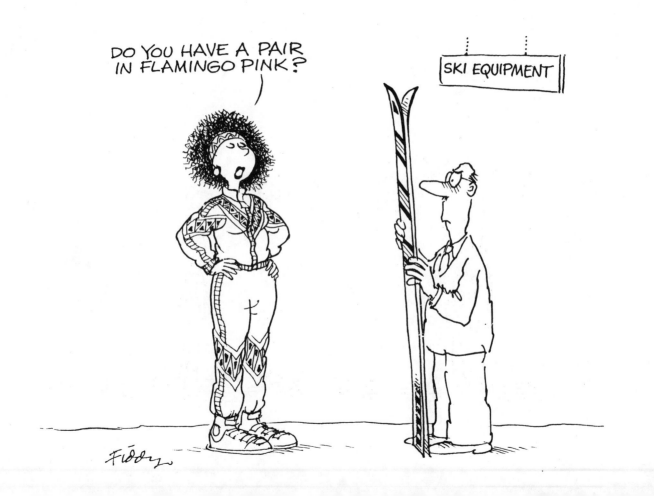

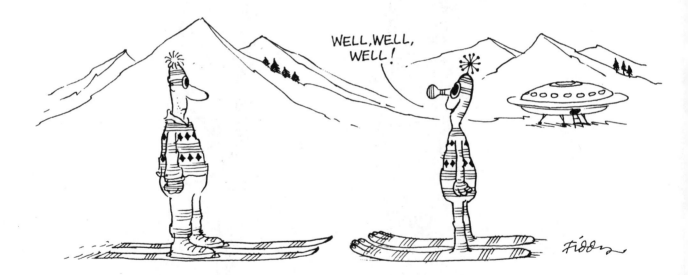

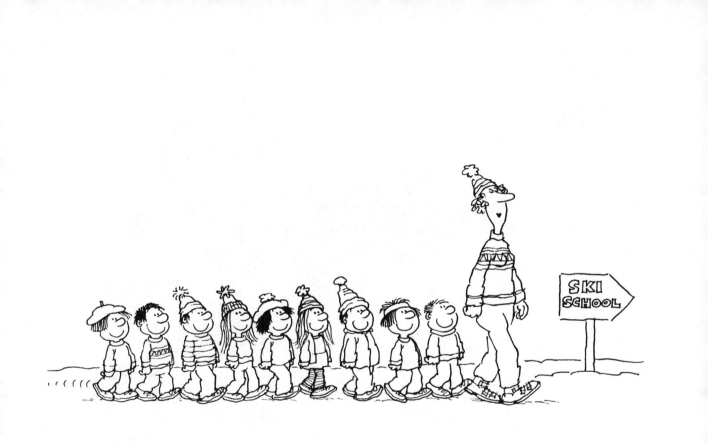

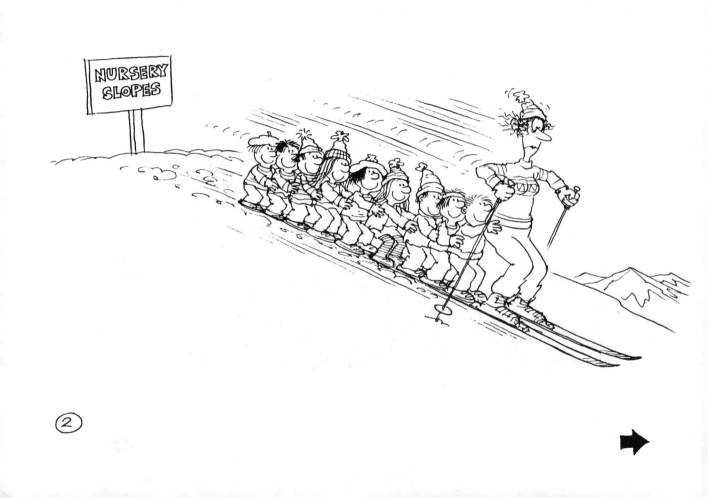

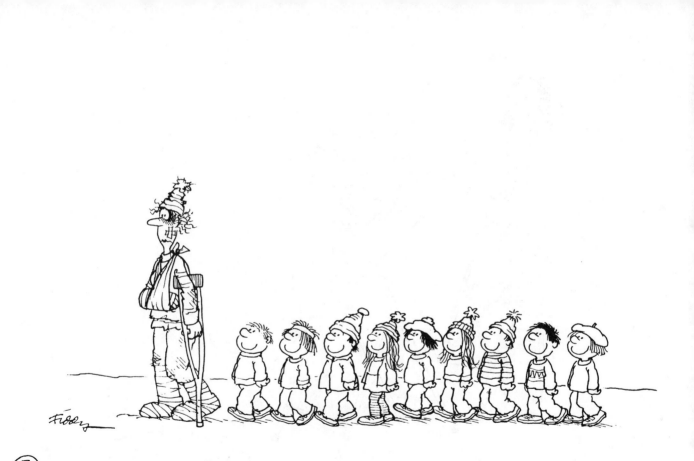

③

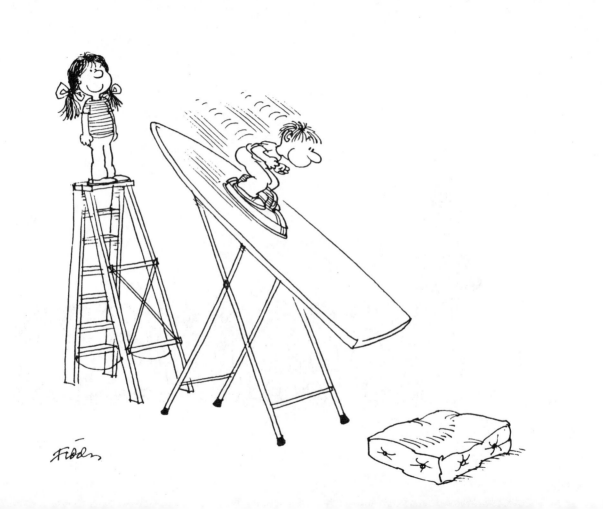

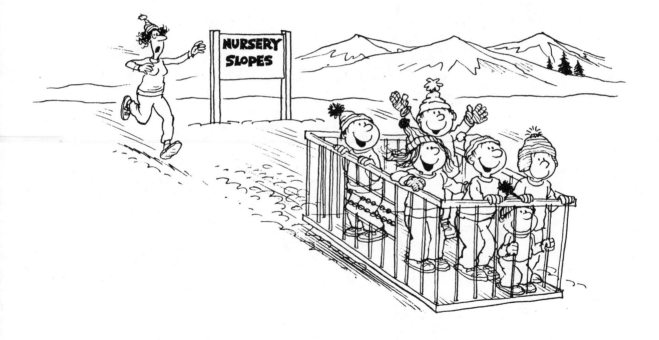

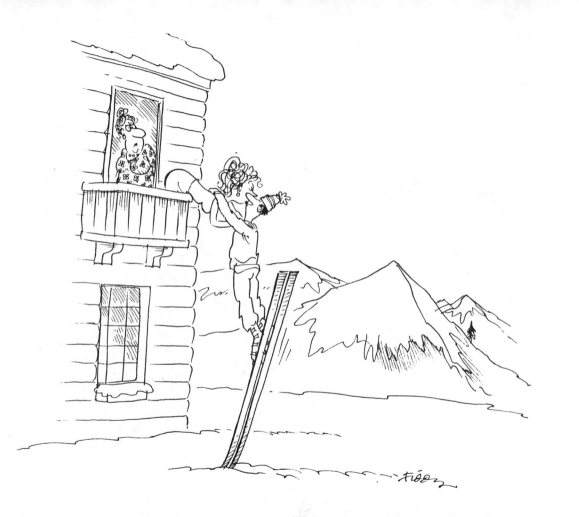

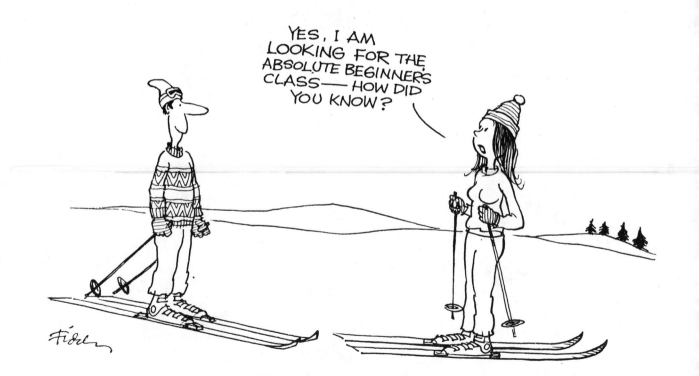

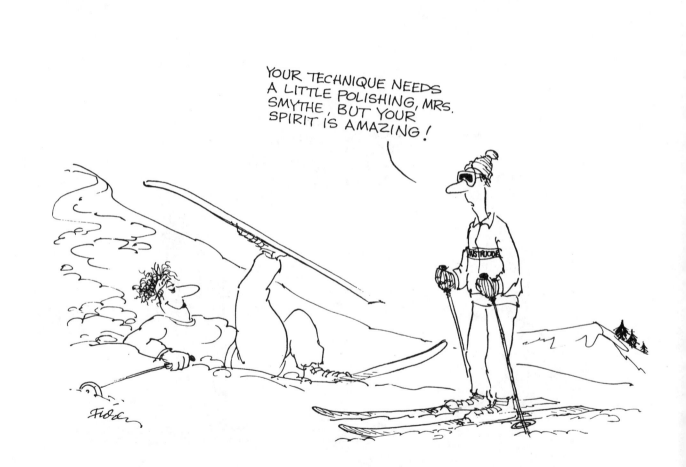

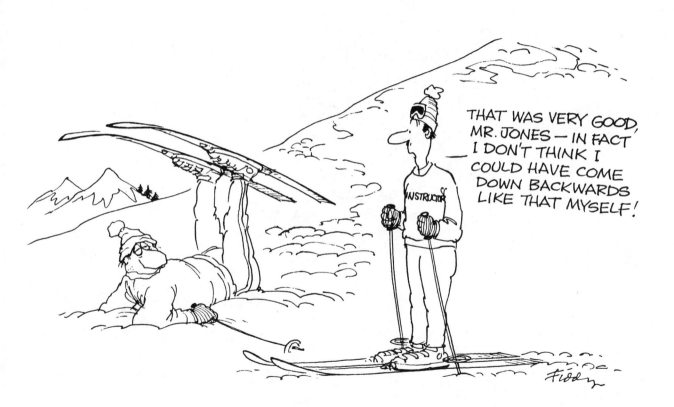

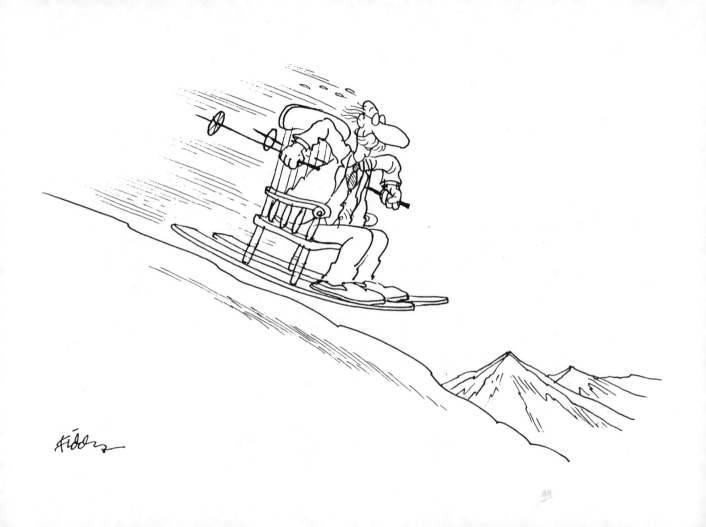

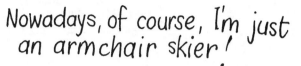
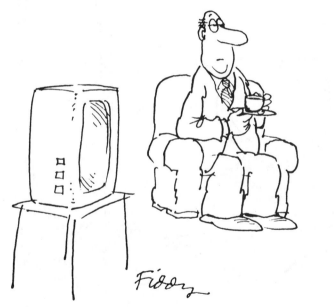
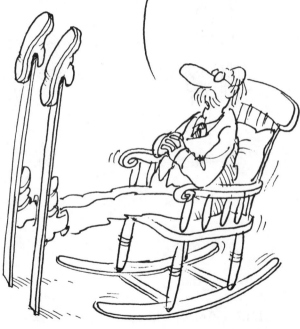

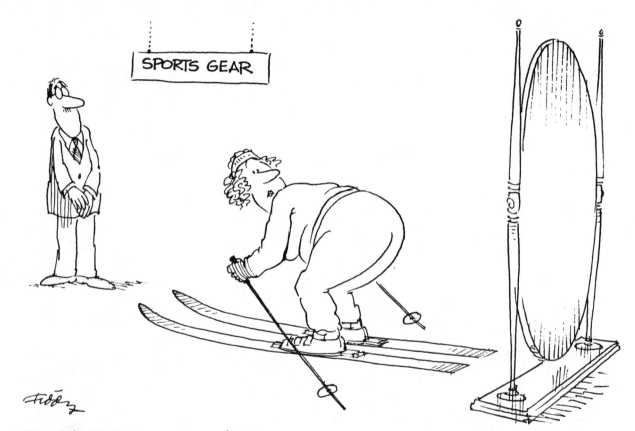

SPORTS GEAR

THE FANATICAL SKIER'S EQUIPMENT IS CHOSEN WITH CARE....

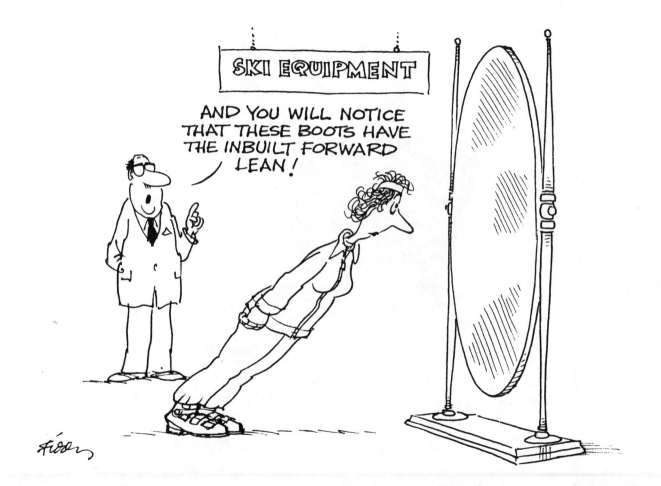

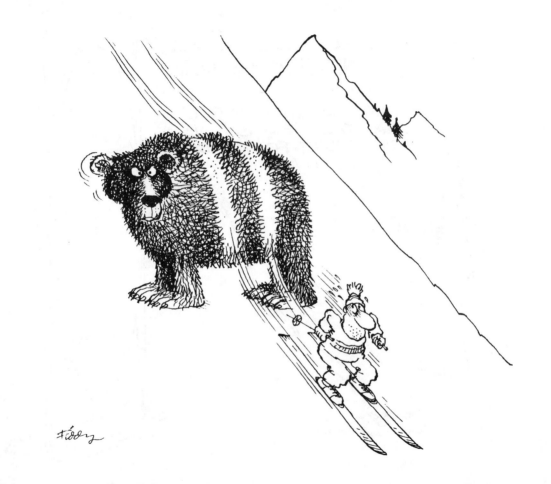

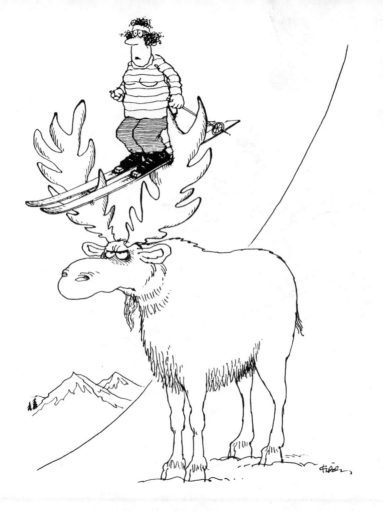

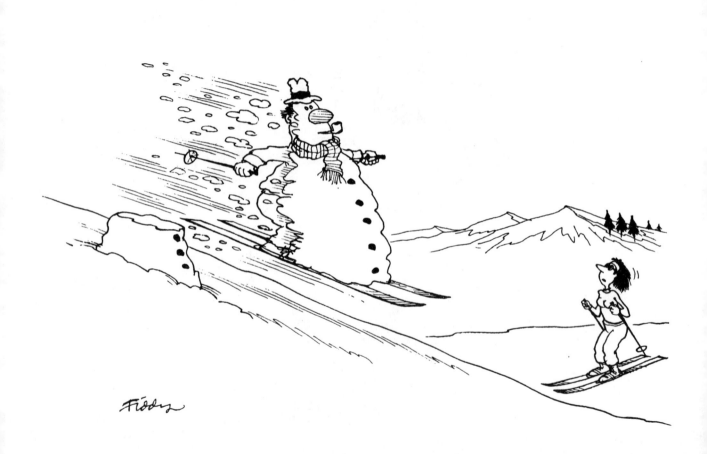

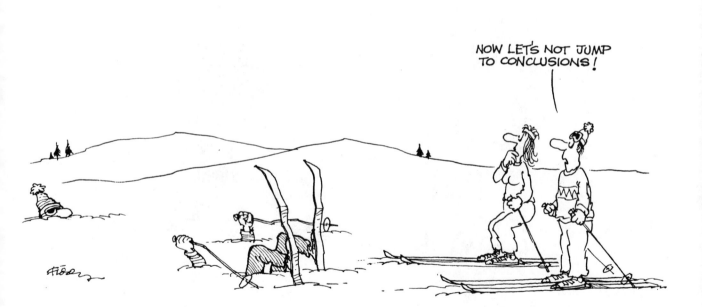

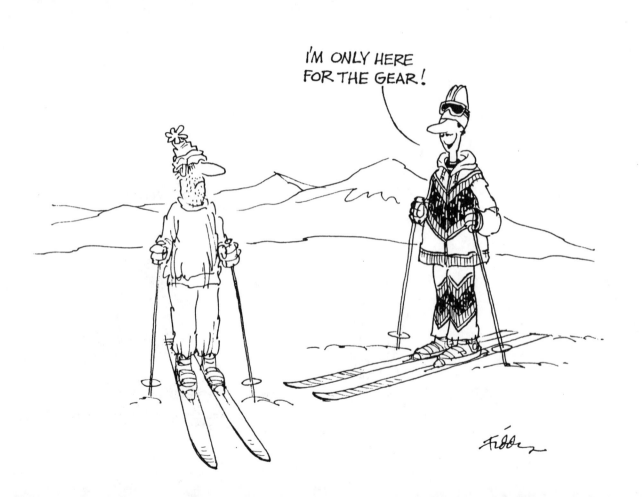

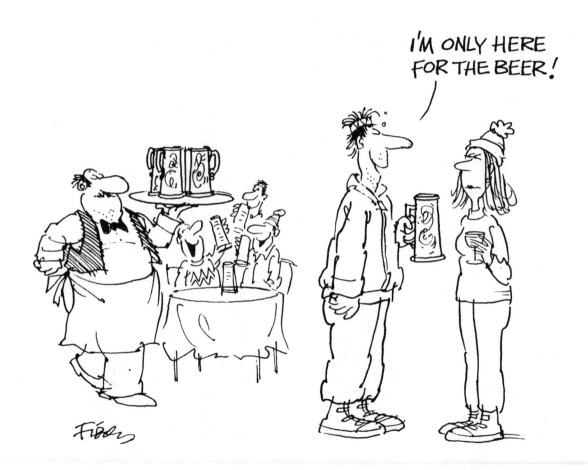

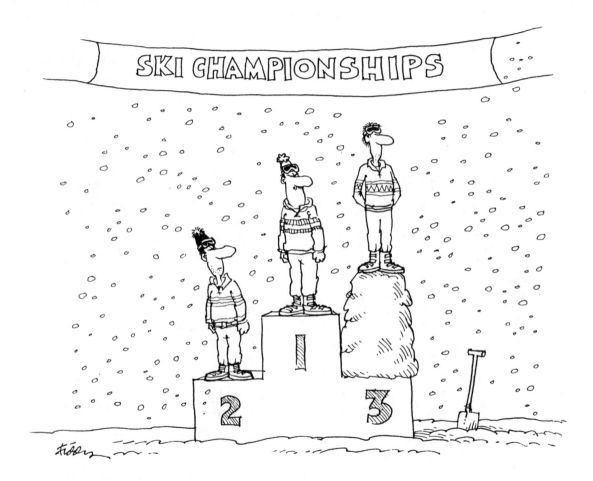

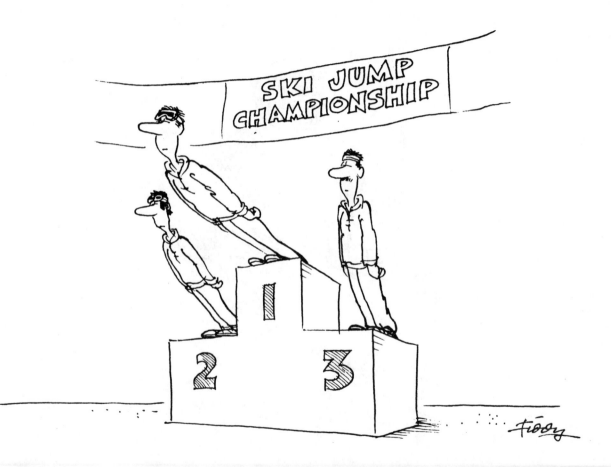

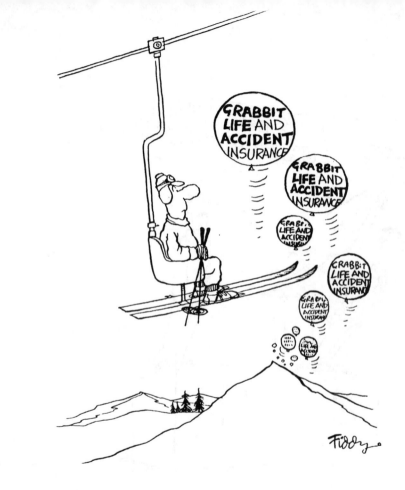

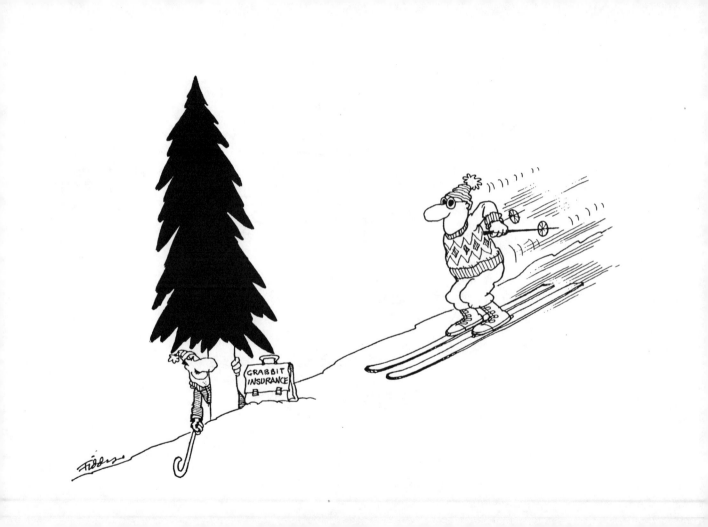

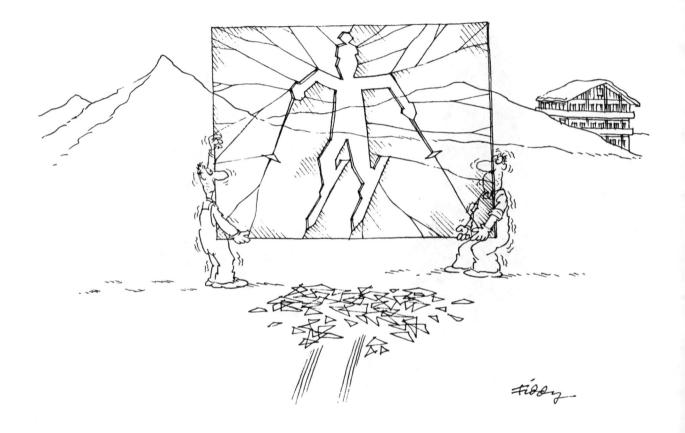

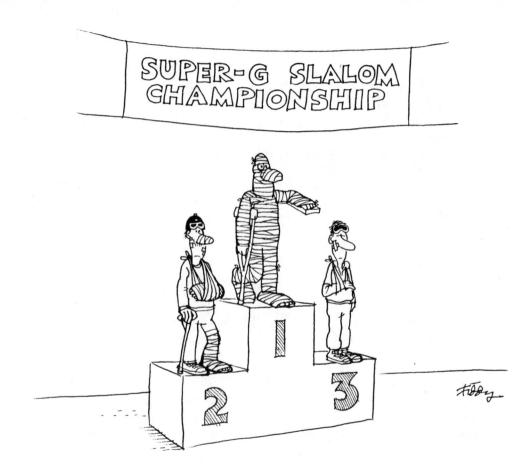

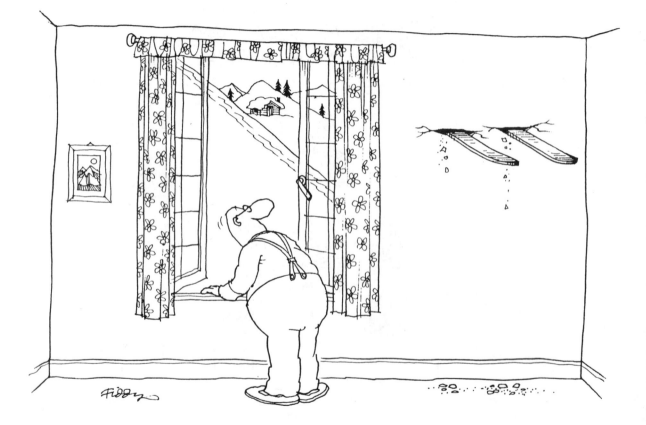

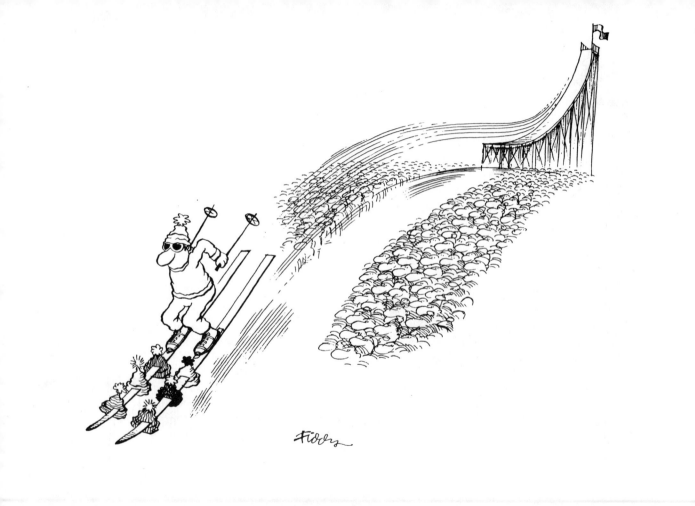

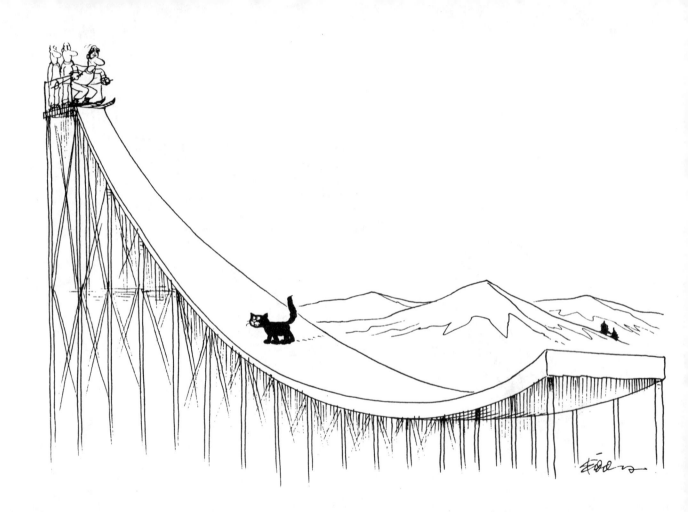

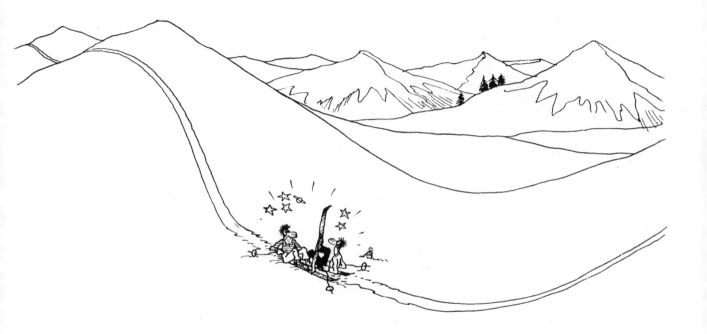

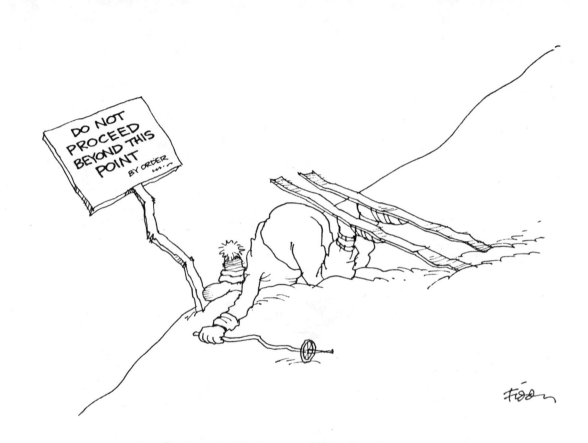

FANATICAL SKIERS MUST OBEY THE SIGNS .

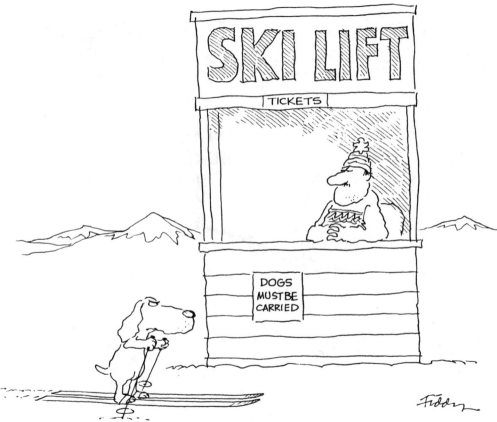

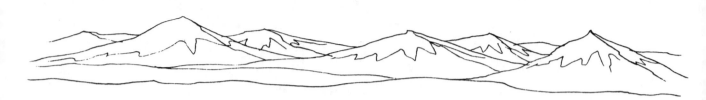
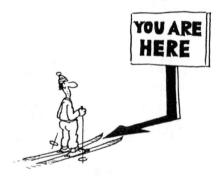

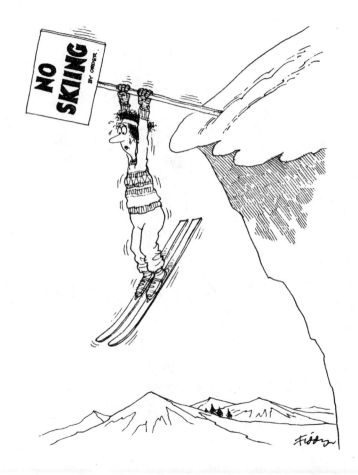

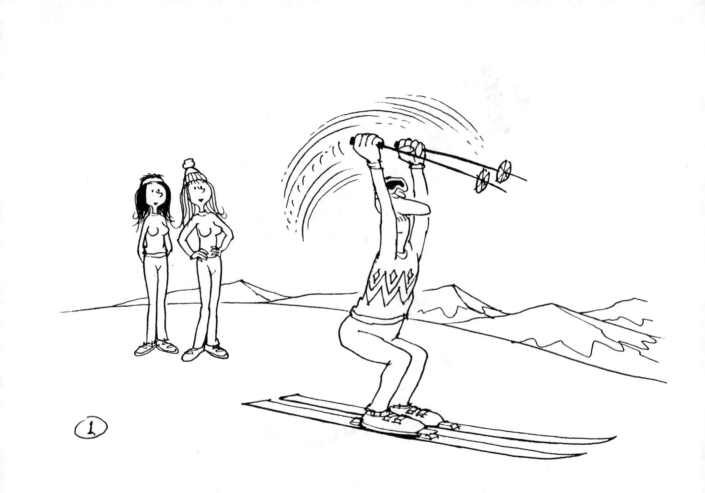

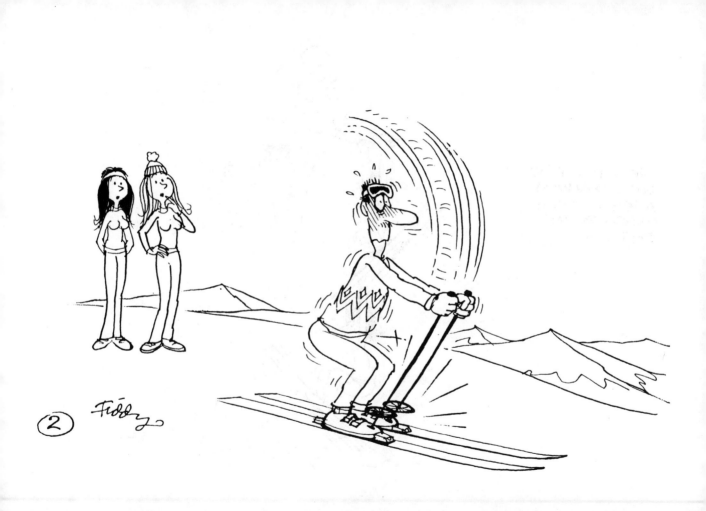

THE SKIING FANATIC
SHOULD ALWAYS
ASSIST OTHERS
WHO ARE IN
DIFFICULTY....

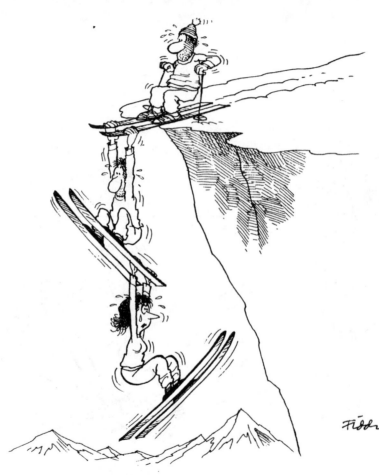

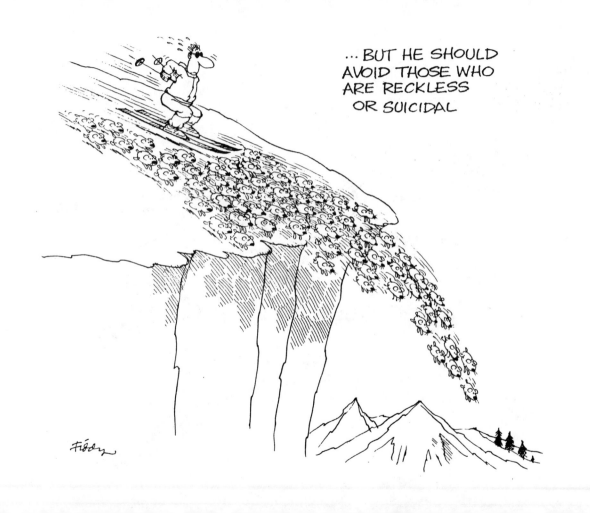

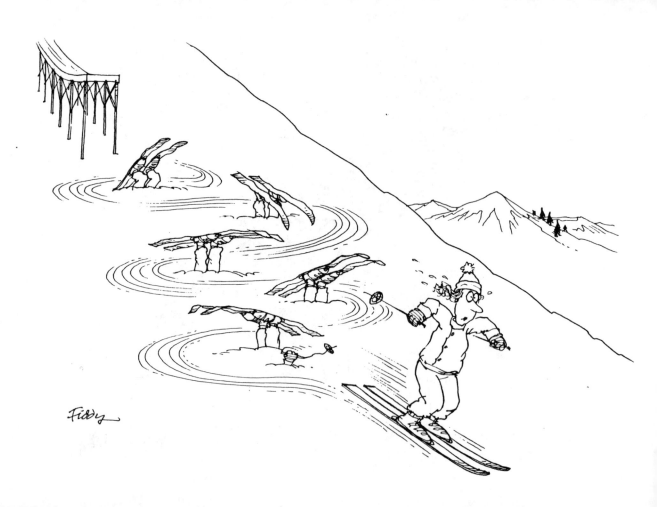

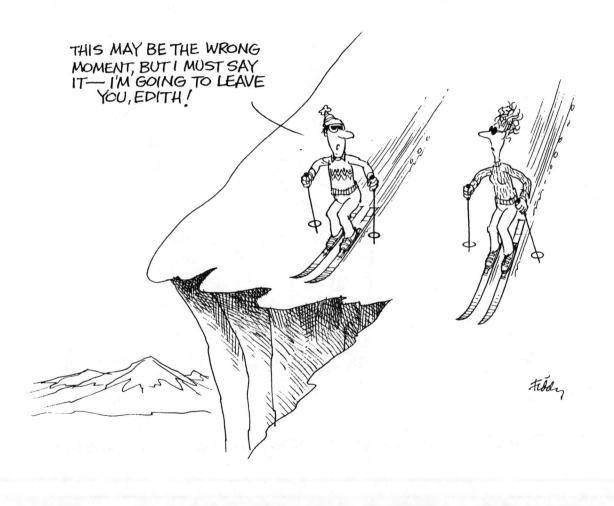

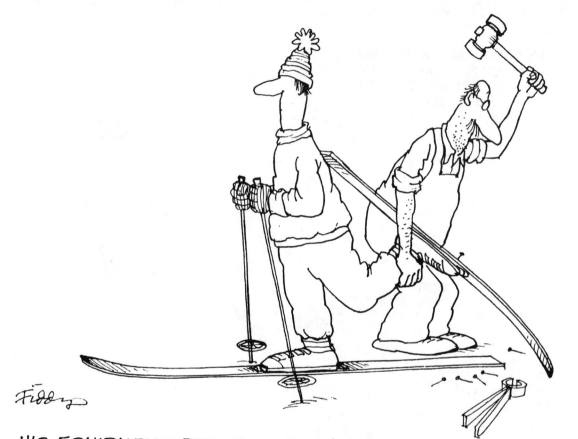

HIS EQUIPMENT BECOMES ALMOST A PART OF HIMSELF

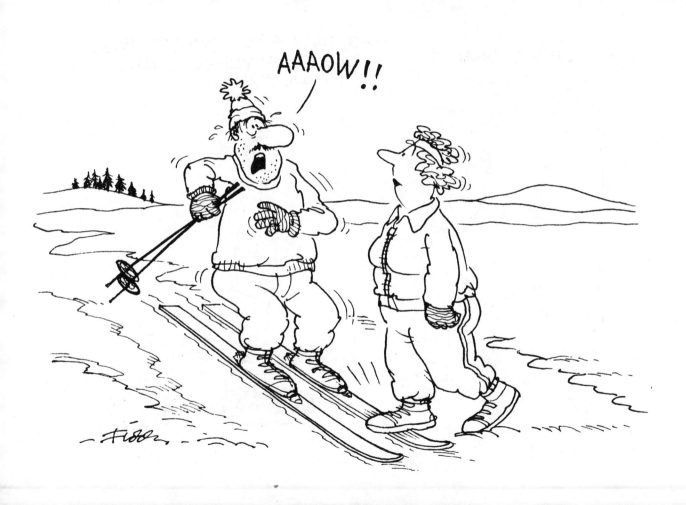

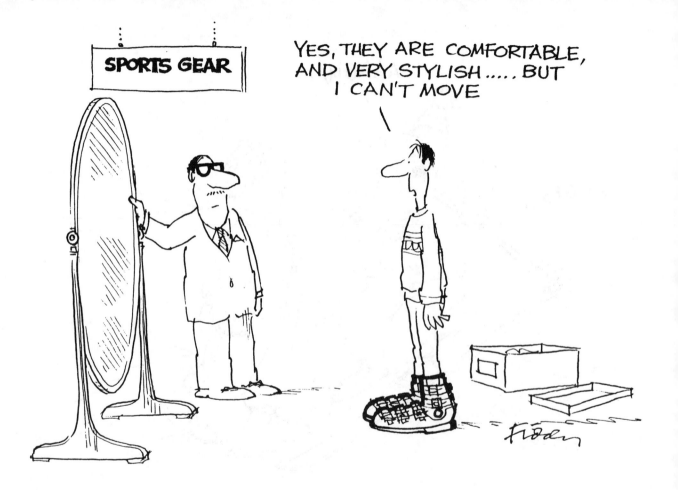

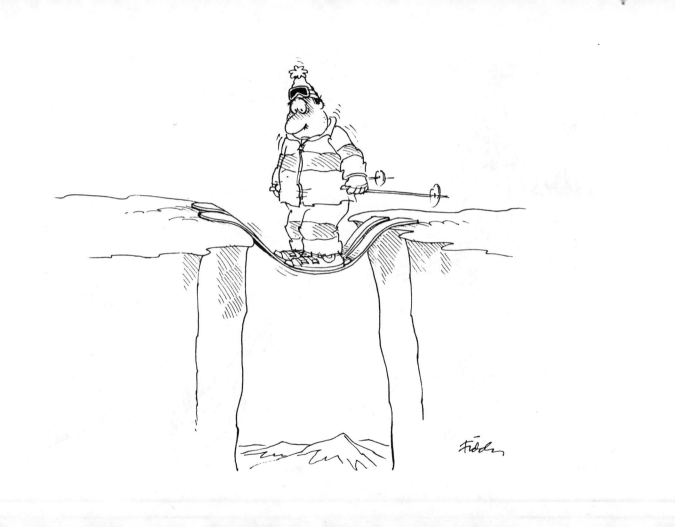

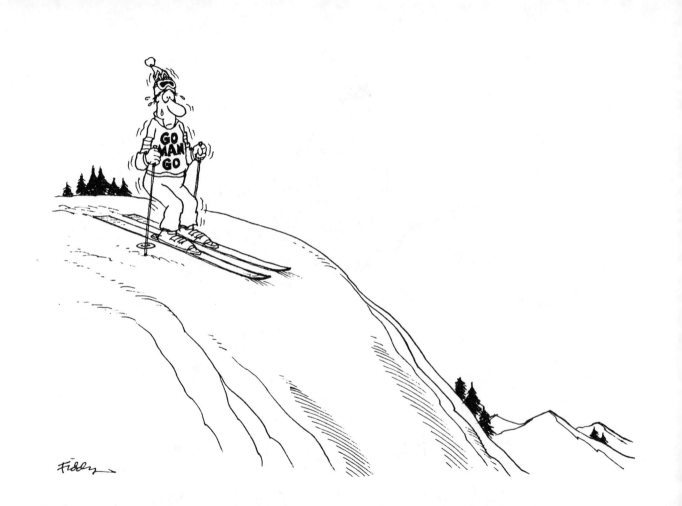

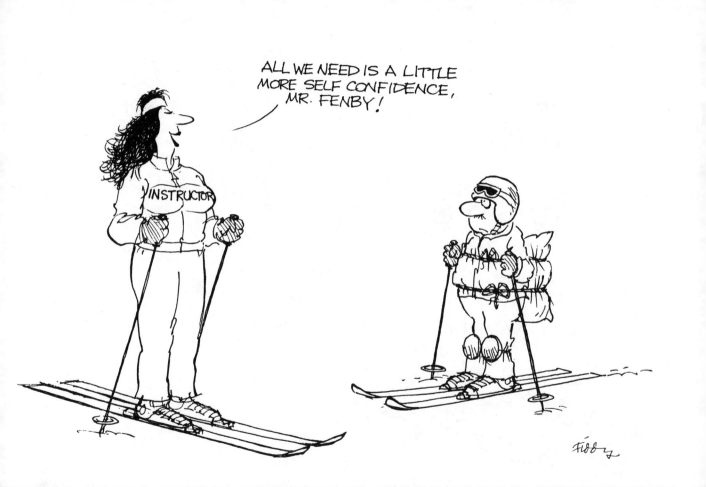

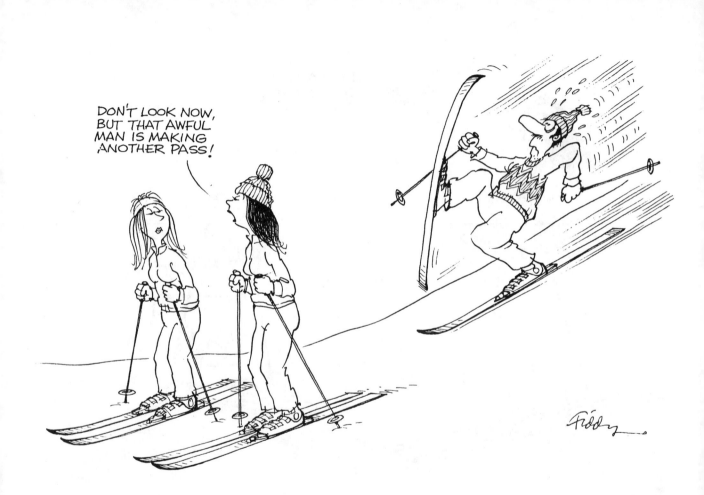

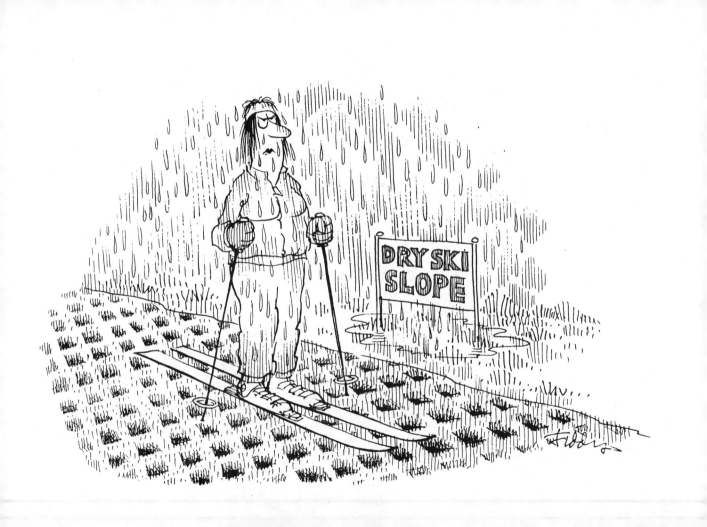

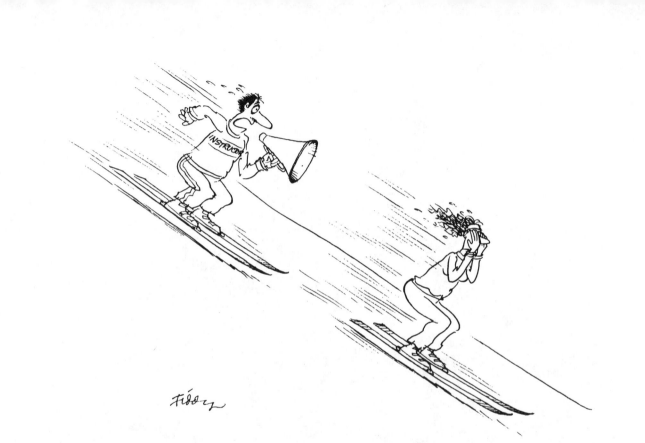

WHEN SKIING IT IS ESSENTIAL TO KEEP **ALL** ONE'S SENSES ALERT.

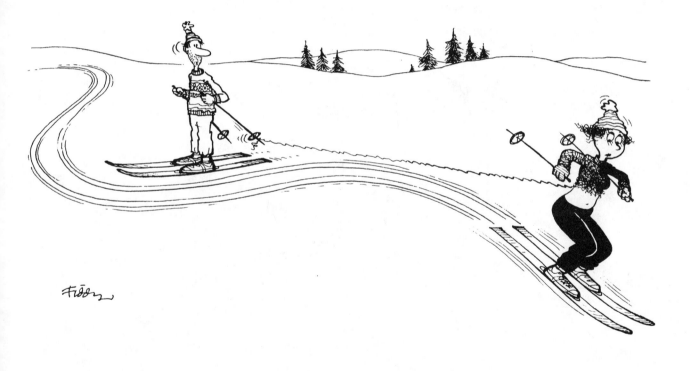

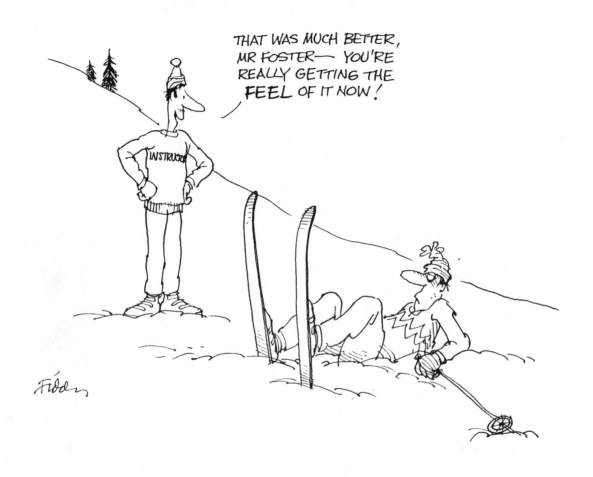

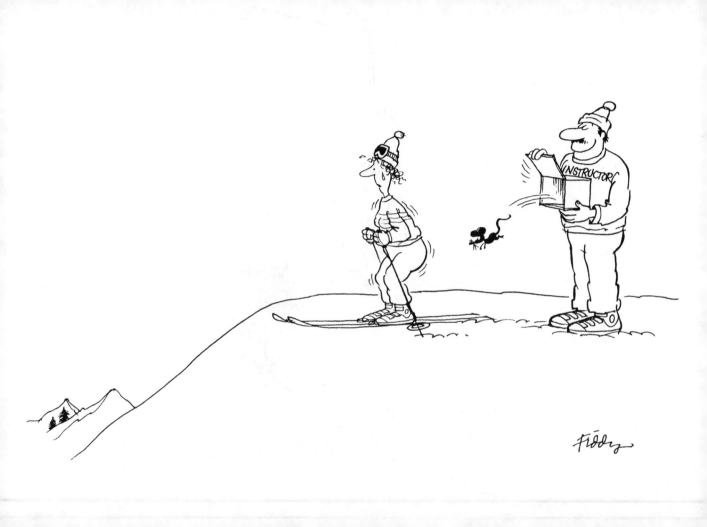

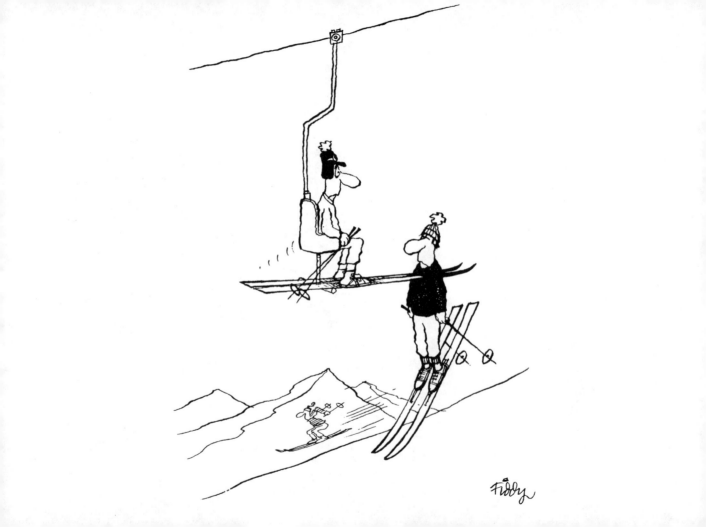

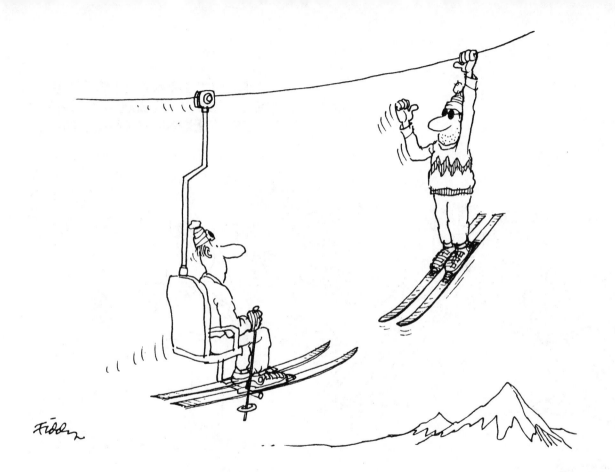

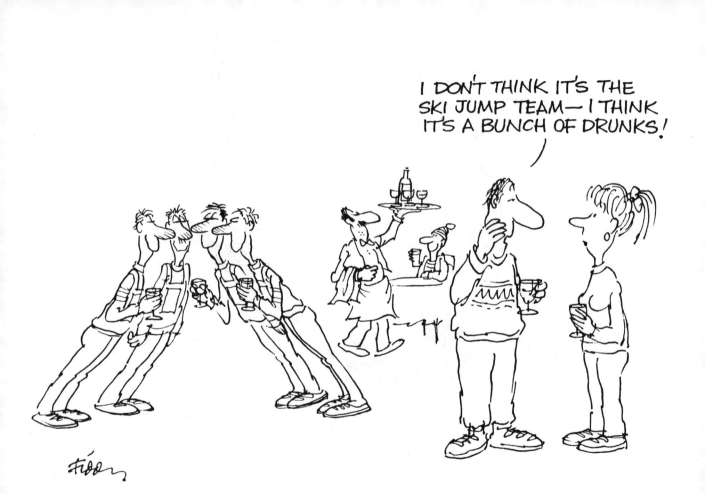

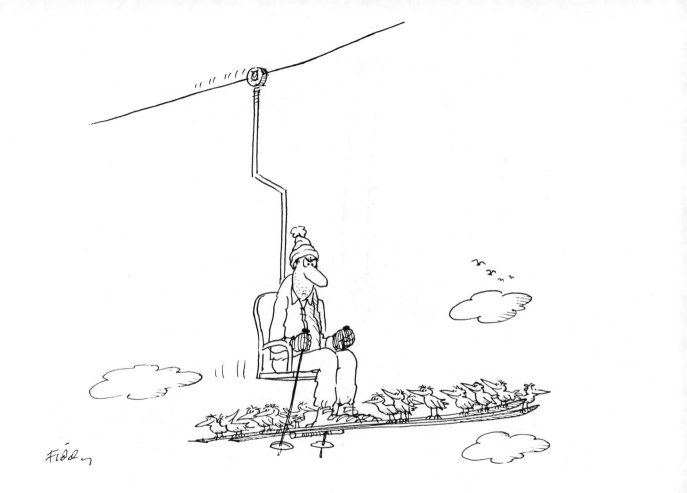

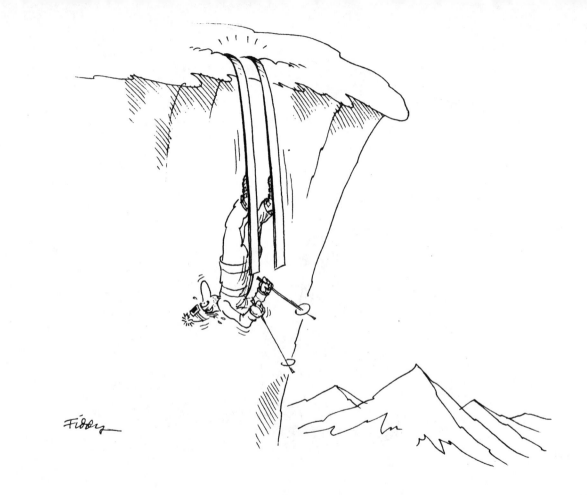

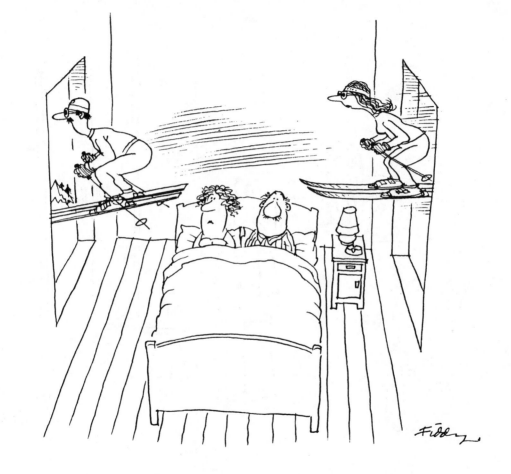

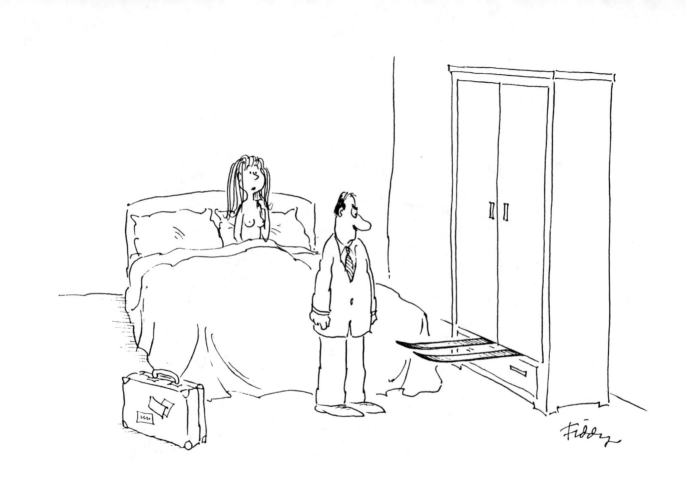

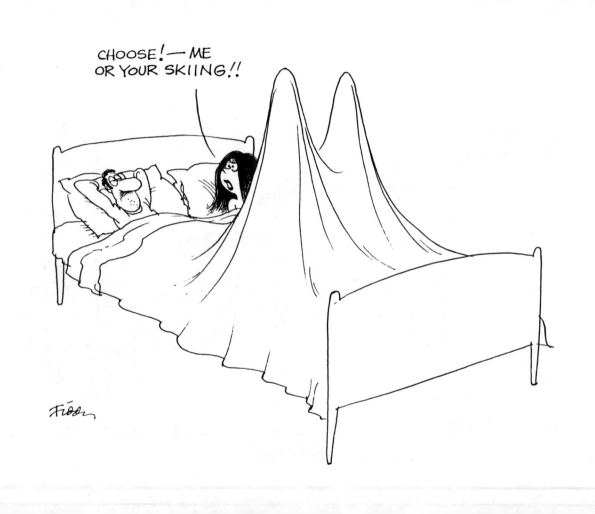

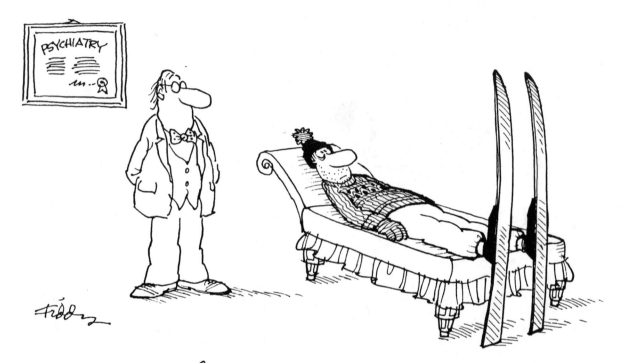

A SKI-ZOPHRENIC (one who can't bear to be parted from his skis for a moment)

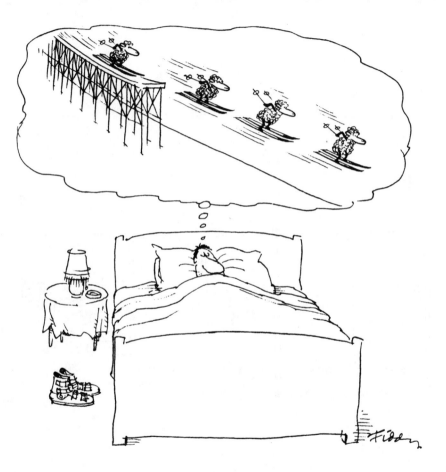

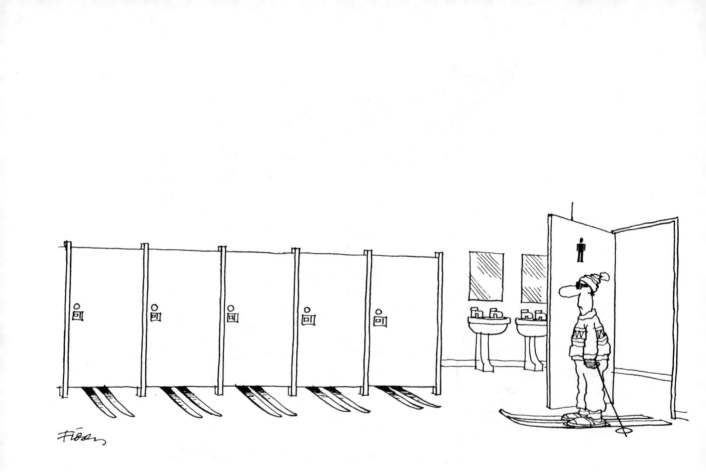

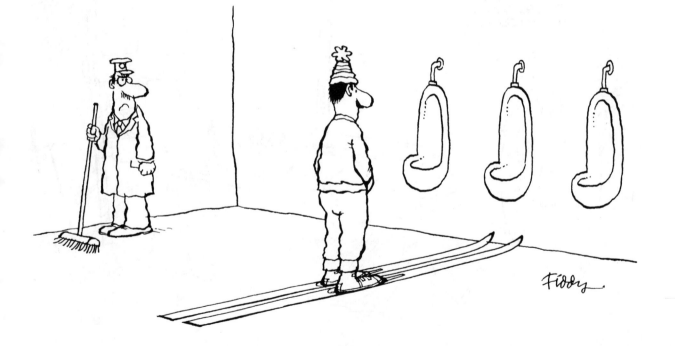

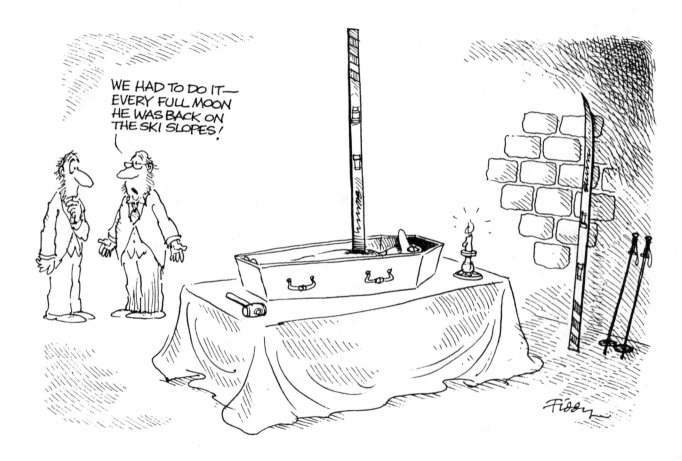

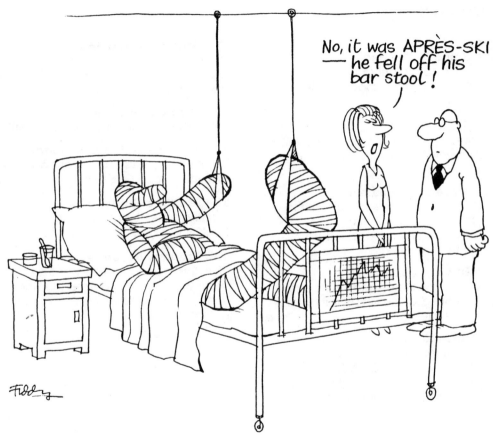

Cartoons by Roland Fiddy

The Crazy World series

There are now 20 different titles in this best selling cartoon series – one of them must be right for a friend of yours....

The Crazy World of Birdwatching (Peter Rigby)
The Crazy World of Cats (Bill Stott)
The Crazy World of Cricket (Bill Stott)
The Crazy World of Gardening (Bill Stott)
The Crazy World of Golf (Mike Scott)
The Crazy World of the Handyman
  (Roland Fiddy)
The Crazy World of Hospitals (Bill Stott)
The Crazy World of Jogging (David Pye)
The Crazy World of Love (Roland Fiddy)
The Crazy World of Marriage (Bill Stott)
The Crazy World of Music (Bill Stott)
The Crazy World of the Office (Bill Stott)
The Crazy World of Photography (Bill Stott)
The Crazy World of the Royals (Barry Knowles)
The Crazy World of Rugby (Bill Stott)
The Crazy World of Sailing (Peter Rigby)
The Crazy World of the School (Bill Stott)
The Crazy World of Sex (David Pye)
The Crazy World of Skiing
  (Craig Peterson & Jerry Emerson)
The Crazy World of Tennis (Peter Rigby)

Great Britain: Order these super books from your local bookseller or from Exley Publications Ltd, 16 Chalk Hill, Watford, Herts WD1 4BN. (Please send £1.25 to cover post and packing on 1 book, £2.50 on 2 or more books.)

Roland Fiddy

Roland Fiddy is a freelance cartoonist and illustrator. He was born in Devon in Great Britain. His cartoons have been published in Britain, the United States, Germany, Holland and many other countries, and have received numerous awards at International Cartoon Festivals. At the Knokke-Heist Festival in Belgium in 1990 Roland Fiddy won First Prize, and, more recently, he was awarded the Prize for Excellence at Yomiuri Shimbun, Tokyo in 1991. His published books include all the *Fanatic's Guides* in the Exley series: *The Fanatic's Guide to The Bed, The Fanatic's Guide to Cats, The Fanatic's Guide to Computers, The Fanatic's Guide to Dads, The Fanatic's Guide to Diets, The Fanatic's Guide to Dogs, The Fanatic's Guide to Golf, The Fanatic's Guide to Husbands, The Fanatic's Guide to Money, The Fanatic's Guide to Sex* and *The Fanatic's Guide to Skiing.* He is also the cartoonist of *The Crazy World of the Handyman* and *The Crazy World of Love,* which are both published by Exley.